THIS COSTLY SEASON

A CROWN OF SONNETS

ARROWSMITH
PRESS

This Costly Season
John Okrent

ISBN: 978-1-7376156-5-1

Boston — New York — San Francisco — Baghdad
San Juan — Kyiv — Istanbul — Santiago, Chile
Beijing — Paris — London — Cairo — Madrid
Milan — Melbourne — Jerusalem — Darfur

11 Chestnut St.
Medford, MA 02155

arrowsmithpress@gmail.com
www.arrowsmithpress.com

The fortieth Arrowsmith book
was typeset & designed by Ezra Fox
for Askold Melnyczuk & Alex Johnson
in Baskerville typeface

Cover Image: *Untitled (Cherry Blossoms)*, 2021
© Curran Hatleberg

THIS COSTLY SEASON

JOHN OKRENT

For X & O

Though trees turn bare and girls turn wives,
We shall afford our costly seasons;
There is a gentleness survives
That will outspeak and has its reasons.
There is a loveliness exists,
Preserves us, not for specialists.

– *April Inventory*, W. D. Snodgrass

March 17, 2020

Driving to clinic—on the radio a pulmonologist

in Italy tells of choosing among the dying

which ones not to save. I picture Whitman,

wending his way through wounded Union

soldiers—his democratic nostrils, the smell of dead

or dying flesh. And in all the dooryards, the smell of lilacs.

It was gorgeous today, and marked the fifty-second death

in the Evergreen State. Everyone's eyes seemed wider

above their face masks. Fear lends an urgent sort of beauty

to the days. When he got back to clinic this evening,

Frankie said it was crazy at the gun shop; everyone grabbing

all the ammo, all the guns. "Business has never been better,"

said the man behind the counter, whom I picture

wearing latex gloves the color of lilacs, only darker.

The color of lilacs, only darker—the clouds
that cover the top of Mt. Rainier this evening
like a shroud. Another beautiful day. Disturbing
to see so many people walking the waterfront.
The fish market is closed. The café is closed.
The bar is closed. The daffodils are heedless.
Today, the first death in Tacoma. A woman
in her fifties. Droplets cover me, probably. My neighbor veers.
Conversation grows heavier by the word.
In clinic I don plastic face shield and gown
of goldenrod when seeing a *person*
under investigation. The nights grow quieter.
We no longer hear passenger trains, only freight trains,
and fewer, from our cabin.

March 19, 2020

From our cabin we keep the world.

Home from clinic I throw my clothes

straight in the wash and get in the shower

before I touch my wife and daughter,

which means Xela has to hide her

so Oola doesn't see me when I come in.

What I bring home with me: mortality

and an empty thermos. A hundred and sixty

new positives in King County. Numbers double

by the day and will and from the dresser last week's tulips

bow their purple, ludicrous heads. This may be the end

of irony. The sky again so blue it could break

from blueness. Sterilized, I hug my girls.

In our cabin we keep the world.

We keep the world, the world keeps us,

the way the oceans keep the continents—

nowhere to go now but down, and in.

Friends and family, faces on my phone—

pixelated flesh-tones. Are they choking up?

The familiar cups of their eyes

overflowing? Or is it just a bad connection?

I miss connection—the compassion of hands—the heat

of faces. The sharp curve of new cases

like a sudden middle finger from a fist.

What if we can't withstand this?

Our dog, thank God, tangential as a dream.

I can't wait for a time when I say "this"

and you don't know what I mean.

March 22, 2020

You don't know what I mean but if beauty
is truth, truth beauty, then life is layered
in redundancy. It was fog on fog on fern-moss
this morning when I took my daughter
for a walk in the woods. From the palm
of my hand she picked bits of granola. Corona-
virus has killed its thousands now, and now
its tens of thousands. Two teenage boys
jogged by us on the path; the smell of their deodorant
reminded me of a time when the world was exuberant,
or buoyant, at least. It's sinking in,
this sinking thing. We didn't see another soul all day.
The air felt prehistoric on my naked face.
I shaved my beard so that the mask might fit.

The mask might fit but its breadth is wanting.

I tell my patient he's breathing fine

and has no fever and there aren't enough tests,

enough masks, enough us—I can't test him for the virus.

He coughs. His red socks and black sneakers,

the most articulate image of my day

as he storms from the clinic, rank particulates

scattering and settling on everything.

I never saw his mouth, just his beard below his mask

cascading down his chest—it was beautiful,

even more beautiful than the rainbow I saw later

driving home. Crowds gathered along the water to watch

and somewhere, cornered in their minds, each—of the other—

thinking—beneath their breath: "if you die it is not my death."

March 27, 2020

If you die it is not my death:

our fundamental difference, our distance.

We're discontinuous—or so thought a French philosopher

who was there in 1918 when the Spanish Flu killed hundreds

of thousands of French people. The Spanish Flu, from Kansas,

USA. Pink plastic bags on top of coffins—the belongings

of the dead who were alive today. Alone. Alone,

and everything, even funerals, postponed. And now

my visits are on the phone. In the background, rain and the racket

of TV and dishes. And behind my patient's voice a smaller one,

the president's, insidious, saying he wants the country

open for business by Easter. A ship of empty gurneys

waits at the pier. We must learn to feel the pain of things

that are not yet here. Business for Easter: if you die, I die too.

If you die I die too. I am here for you,

on my lunch break, where the magnolia is encumbered

by the indulgence of spring—rude, decadent

white blossoms. The Department of Health's website

is down today so the dead remain unnumbered.

There's a woman who sleeps in the alley

behind the library near here—I saw her earlier

in a bad way beneath the magnolia tree

and couldn't help her. A directive to the non-essential:

shut down, stay home. But home is luck. And what's essential?

The liquor store, the gas station, the commercial geoduck

operation—there's a lot that's not, a lot that trembles,

like the dandelion I handed Oola in the last of the sun,

wishing fields of yellow flowers, a world like this one.

April 4, 2020

A world like this one, even this one,

will be fine—as in finished, perfected. But I'm

fragmented—and so tired

of the dead. Over a thousand over the weekend

in just New York. And there's talk of temporary

burials in public parks. In Ojai, Nick watches

a show about rival pontiffs on a precipice.

In Paris, Eleanor listens to *Bleak House* and walks

her allotted radius. Cindy and Curran in Baltimore

labor for twenty-four hours, alone, before their baby is born.

They name him River.

It's so hard not to hold one another.

Already the daffodils have shriveled and dried.

Summer will be the death of springtime.

This dying in springtime will reach its "plateau,"

as they call it. Ralph calls it the "piccolo cry"

when the hummingbird calls my attention

and is gone. Ruby-throated dart. *A point*

is that which has no part. A line is breadthless length.

Our geometry is rough; it is muddled by our bodies.

The globe is not a perfect sphere; it is lumpy with the buried.

I was startled by the moon tonight, closer than it will come

all year. A "pink moon," we call it, not because it is,

but for the phlox blooming in the meadows and on the rocks

this time of year. When the days are done, from their isolation

people come to cheer "essential workers," meaning everyone,

all of us, alone together, living—blooming, even,

on this molten rock where, for a billion years, nothing did.

Nothing did, and then something did,

and now it seems there is nothing that is not

flowering. The laurel along the road, the wild

blueberries, the hushed bells of the bearberry bush,

the cherry trees and their tantrums

of white blossoms as the dead are wheeled beneath them

covered in white sheets. Easter morning. A plastic egg

on the front porch for Oola. I toss the candy

when she turns away and fill it with pebbles. It's the rattle

that pleases her anyway. The way she says *Easter*

it sounds like *eaten*. The madrones look like dancers' arms

reaching from the earth. *This is my body, broken for you,*

said Jesus. "I love you. I miss you. This will end,"

I said to my friend, and almost meant it.

I almost meant it, but meaning is refracted—

sunlight through a pill bottle on the sill.

Yellow pollen on my windshield

like confetti from a sorority party

at a college whose mascot's a canary. I could not describe

the smell of the cherry-laurel blossoms to my sister

so I said they smelled yellow, like the yellow flower dress

she yearned for as a kid—*well woe, fouler duress.* I call her

every evening on my way home from clinic and tell her

what I see, not saw: a woman in a mask straddling a man

in a mask on a bench, a woman with no arms or legs

on a skateboard, tiny archers at the edge of the woods

and, when I pull into the parking lot, two kids

on pogo sticks, laughing, like gravity is the joke.

April 16, 2020

Gravity is a joke to the cherry blossoms

which turn the trees to cumulus clouds

loosely tethered to the earth. This will serve

as the forum for our doldrums. Much of the world

in pajamas. Warehouse full of superfluous

pants. My dog sniffs a feather in the grass

and maybe it fires some forgotten synapse—a flash

of flight. More likely, his teeth gleam remembering

the taste of fowl. The sky smells like ozone. This resists

the imagination. *Ozone*, from the ancient Greek,

Ozein: to smell. Sky blue sky. *You are entering the medical record*

of a patient who has died—red letters alert me from the screen.

The red of the rhododendrons this spring—like a warning

passed down through the centuries, urgently.

Over centuries, urgently, we learned

to stand up and walk but tonight I want to fall

down and stay there—something like prayer.

I don't believe in progress. The days keep falling

like bricks from rushed construction. All night

it rained and this morning the water was the opaque color

of a newborn's eyes. Sheet-metal clouds make it easy

to stay inside. Maybe fewer will die. A Spanaway man

in his forties. "We're going to open it up in beautiful little pieces,"

says the president and I picture the carcass of a rhinoceros

but he means the country. A Bonney Lake man in his sixties.

Oola stands and walks on knees as wobbly as a foal's.

Her small feet grip the spinning globe. First steps in every pasture,

calf hoof and lamb—faint vibrations in the ear—that time of year.

April 20, 2020

That time of year when every crow you see

carries clump of hair or twig or tuft of down

into the trees. They brood and hover

over our duress while spring repays last summer's

debts. "We shall afford our costly seasons," said Snodgrass.

But this one? Like a stain, desperation seeps into things:

the grocery bag, the steering wheel, little hand

in my hand, midnight bowl of cereal.

Before leaving for clinic I toss my daughter

high and higher into the faultless air

like any father. Later, with soap and water

I'll wash the formless fruits of my labor.

The mist hangs low around the whole horizon

like the lid of an eye that's closing. But it's only morning.

It's only morning but I am ready

for bed, for dinner, a drink, the dark

horizon pearled with lit rooms. I admit it,

I've grown used to being alive.

And I'm tired, already, of this poem—

of the *I* in it. In the parking lot in her yellow gown

Ana reaches a swab through the window of a car

and up the driver's nose until he gags. Beyond this, brown

birds on municipal wires, chartreuse of spring on the trees,

trash bags in the alleys, American flags sagging

from the eaves. It's a summer flag if ever there was one,

which reminds me: summer will come, despite us.

I bow my head to the gun

of the infrared thermometer, then enter the clinic.

I enter the clinic and come closer to others

than most others can come these furrowed days,

days at once so full of distance and congestion—

a person could choke on air. And people do. Cerulean blue

and rococo clouds above the I-5 corridor:

the largesse of the here and now.

Small comforts stretch to compensate our largest fear.

Purell dispensers on the plastered walls

like primitive masks with tragic frowns. Squirt,

squirt. I can feel that something hurts but don't know how

or even in whose body. Wild poppies on the side of the road

like tiny monks in their saffron robes. From a distance

I thought the fire hydrant was a crucifix

and marked a grave. How many ways can a man be saved?

Two blocks from clinic, every morning, to be saved

I pass the same cloister of chain-link and small trees

whose blossoms take a deeper shade of fuchsia by the day.

A woman always lets her dogs out then. She smokes

and leans in her robe. Her shower-cap is the same fuchsia

as the blossoms. Her Chihuahua crouches to shit and she leaves it.

The light turns, and I roll on. The earth holds almost all

we think is gone. When Oola laughs in her sleep

I wonder, what are dreams to one so newly here? These evenings

on our walks I press her nose to lilacs and exaggerate delight

as if, breathing thus, we might transcend. We are made of breathing

and breathing ends. But we are also made of dust, which doesn't.

The air is warm tonight, and barely there, like a memory of being

touched. Life isn't fair—it's beautiful.

May 5, 2020

It is beautiful to be glad to see a person

every time you see them, as I was to see Juan,

the maintenance man, with whom it was always the same

brotherly greeting—each of us thumping a fist

over his heart and grinning, as though we shared a joke,

or bread. I barely knew him. Evenings in clinic,

me finishing my work, him beginning his—

fluorescence softening in the early dark. He wasn't even fifty,

had four grandchildren, fixed what was broken, cleaned

for us, caught the virus, and died on his couch

last weekend. And what right have I to write this poem,

who will not see him in his uniform of ashes,

only remember him, in his Seahawks cap, and far from sick,

locking up after me, turning up his music.

His music he no longer hears, his hands,

hardly hands—little lines of personhood

erased—no longer grip or trace

the day's detritus with a mop. So long, Juan.

We will perform the daily miracle of moving on

without semblance of touch, in this unseasonable

warmth, mingle our particular molecules, enter

one another even—rain falling into fog.

Oola's grandfather has been writing songs.

When he plays them for her on the phone,

her reaching is so fervent it tips her over,

as though his voice alone could catch and hold her.

I refuse to get used to these disembodied ways. I want

to wrap my arms around the days, to kiss their drooping shoulders.

May 18, 2020

Drooping shoulders demonstrate how grief

overflows its soft containers. It runs down arms

and falls from fingers and pools at the feet

of the couple, for example, taking up their bed

from the sidewalk, and the woman at the bus stop

not getting on, and the man

turning racks of ribs at the bar-b-q spot, just open

after two months shut—smoke pours from his grill

and obscures the cross, Christ nailed on the kitchen wall.

To inherit the earth is to inherit loss.

Forty years ago today and seventy miles south

Mount St. Helens blew, killing birds and deer and bear by the thousand

and at least fifty-seven people, one of whom ran from the blast

a few miles before he fell, drowned in the air turned ash.

The ash turned earth, the earth turned grass

and the musk ox grazed it while we watched

from the perimeter of the zoo closed since March.

Memorial Day weekend and everyone out is in

a mask—their eyes like tired swimmers come up for air

with gasps. Oola reaches for my mask

and babbles: *max, max ox, muck ox, max off.*

U.S. DEATHS NEAR 100,000, AN INCALCULABLE LOSS

I can only read ten of their names before reaching

for abstraction. The musk ox hangs its impossible

head. Even the duck tucks its bill under wing

and sleeps. But look up: small birds breach the everywhere

surface of the air, sing, and want nothing.

Sing and want nothing, I say to myself
as I walk in the woods with my daughter.
Incongruous date that commemorates
the dead and the beginning of summer—
the mood is grey this Memorial Day
and the rain doesn't fall so much as prick
the air at the edge of my face. *My face!*
My face! I screamed, fifteen springs past,
emerging thrilled from an unfrozen river.
Being young was nothing but intimacy
with beginning. But the world is older than ever now
and Oola wants to touch each tree, so we move slowly
through the centuries of trunks,
her small voice demanding: *more touch, more touch.*

More touch, more treasure, more muscular mothers

pleasured at peace, more tender our fathers, more police

without weapons but flowers in their teeth, more flaccid

the powers that be, more placid the hours, more love-

tangled sheets, more sun on the floor, more lingering over

the underwear drawer, more offerings burned, more fire

unfurled, more unclutching of pearls, more strangers,

more strangeness, more worlds in the world, more gentle,

more genital, more wrestling with angels, more asphyxia's opposite,

more rest on the mountain, more view from the top of it,

more praying God test me, more saying at daybreak

I will not let you go unless you bless me, more breaking, more open,

more battered my heart, more friction, more spark, more seeing

in the dark. It will get darker. More dark.

June 5, 2020

More dark, my comfort. Leafy green. I know nothing.

The moon is full tonight but I can't see it. Night clouds

redouble the dark and the lights on the bridge are lethargic.

Our dog is on steroids. It's very American. We let him out

to piss on the hour. He breathes in his sleep as if purging.

Tomorrow there's a march across the bridge

with Black Lives Matter and Mothers Against

Police Brutality. "Chest pain with activity

as well as at rest," says pretty much every one

of my patients. I have no idea what all of this is doing to love.

Today I watched a video from a city we used to call home—

a skinny old man, tall as a stop sign, pushed down by cops

in riot gear. The back of his head broke his fall and he lay there

as blood leaked like a secret from his ear.

From the ear, to please the muses, music

reaches for more music. There is dancing today

because it is raining, and that goldfinch on the feeder

is the most vivid thing on two legs. I am listening

to the high tide on the pilings. The wide cups

of the calla lilies are filling with rain.

If I'm not missing someone I'm missing someone else.

Today we got tested, spiraled the self-

swabs up our nostrils in a Walgreens back alley

and passed them back through the crack

in the window. Four hours later, confident

in negatives and stomaching our doubts, we drove south

to see family for the first time in months (our logic

is love-flawed) in that city named for the seat of the gods.

June 10, 2020

The gods sit on us—or they recline,

diaphanous and blind as far as we are concerned.

The closest I've come to believing in God

was when I walked the dry riverbed and heard water.

It was wind in the aspens. What happens

when we find out we haven't even begun?

America, you had one job: feed everyone.

Now even your trees are hungry

and your children wait with singing stomachs

for the bus that brings bologna on white bread,

juice boxes, sad grapes, and apple slices

browning with sweetness. The country is creeping

back open. Like a door in a horror movie.

We've seen this before.

We've seen before we open our eyes

if knowledge is only recollection.

I won't bore you with my dreams—

they're like yours, which is to say:

soundless. Days it rains like this

the bird-feeders are frenetic. I've just been

sitting here willing the sky to stay grey,

the sun to stay gone—that's the level

I'm vibrating on. People think of time as money

but they're wrong. I am trying to be generous

as this stillness that lets everything breathe.

Dust motes dance in the struggling light.

A poppy opens along the path—slowly, then suddenly,

like a heart attack. Time isn't money. Time's what we can't take back.

June 16, 2020

You can't take back the past, it just keeps on
getting larger; regretting is the cost of living
farther. The moose that accordioned our family
car in '86 did something similar to all future
cars. The first woodstove burn left a scar
that has stretched to fit my arm. My first word:
"hot," a warning. Freedom was later, running.
Fast was relative to being caught and no one
tried to catch me. The summer grass was blue
those nights and glad beneath my feet to know me.
Adults and house lights faded like morning stars
and tomorrow hung like a half-moon in the sky
almost as it does today—though not so sadly—
where I can't imagine one more day, let alone July.

Let alone a temperate season,

I forfeit all my expectations. I can't imagine

peaches, let alone plums, let alone sharing them

with friends on a blanket in the grass in the sun,

unmasked and done with the clenched decorum

of this contagion. The sky is an empty stadium

above all the empty stadiums. I can hear in my head

the roar of the crowd like the sound of the sea

in a shell. People are leaving forever

without farewells. How long will I keep mistaking grief

for grace, sympathy for love? I want the precision

of thirst but it hurts to be so thirsty.

I track the worry lines on the faces of my friends

to pools of silence. I can almost drink them.

June 29, 2020

That we drink from the same cup

or share the air

could kill us

or some more fragile someone

we might love.

Things get awfully terrible come Tuesdays

in these warm and eager weeks

where they are busy inventing the future,

forging currency, and teaching us to look

away more quickly. Tonight

I fix my gaze on the dark water

out my window, the barge going by, its bow light

the sort of green that gives permission

—will I miss this when I'm gone?

When I'm gone, no more going on

without news of love, or less. New deaths

like cherries filling up the trees—

dark baubles. Happy Birthday, America,

you are so beautiful and doomed.

In Muckleshoot the fairgrounds are packed

with firework vendors, nuclear families

milling about like gloomy militiamen

in a field of car parts and sparklers,

little fires starting up. There's a secret loneliness

each of us bears and that is our devotion.

The official displays are cancelled this year. Still,

red and green explosions

take tendril-hold on the sky.

From the sky the clouds lower

their dimly-colored udders. We could almost be

in the land of milk and honey. So why do I feel

so down? In an open field, nothing urgent.

I am cradled in the long-lashed gaze

of some Guernsey cows. They are tender

as distant mothers. We are on an island

in the Salish Sea. But the day we came

a humpback whale was struck by our ferry

and sunk, in its endless humility,

away from us. This morning I read the true tally

of this sort of casualty is likely much higher

than we think. Evidence of a strike often sinks,

unwitnessed, never to surface.

July 18, 2020

"Where does the wag go?"
                    -Rebecca Okrent

Never to surface. That's how it is

with the lively dead: we watch them drown in days

that won't stop rising. Today we euthanized our dog.

And by today I don't mean this one but another

now distant enough that I can write it: he is dead.

And now this worried time is worse, and by worse

I mean it feels like war, down to the smallest

particular. The night before, I masked in butter

the pain pill he would not take. And still he wouldn't.

I had to force it in. And it went with him.

Now I remember how he used to sit and watch me

for my better self, or stop with me along the path

to track some scent I couldn't on the air.

I followed my dog into wordlessness, and he left me there.

July 26, 2020

He left me there—here—where I'd rather be

that woman smoking morning cigarettes on her porch

than this man biking to work in the rain. I am waiting

for the epiphany that shows me the world as it is:

suspended, midair, like the button on the shirt

of the man on the bus that has suddenly bounced,

or the waitress who hovered over the outdoor seating

at the Mexican restaurant in that getaway town

and warned us, "Mondays are the new Sundays

now that the tech people have nowhere they have

to be," and when she said, "tech people,"

I pictured the human shapes in those renderings

of amusement parks or stadiums—but I know they are real,

will die, as I will, and that, because of this, nothing is diminished.

Nothing is diminished; even the extinguished

stars still shine so brightly I can't sleep. So late

on a Monday night it is Tuesday morning.

Beside me, my wife and daughter lie still

as houses in a snowy field, and inside them

like candles on a distant windowsill

their dreams are flickering. Today I saw a woman picking

blackberries along the freeway. A small boy, maybe

her son, stood guard, staring down the passing cars.

These days I see desperation in the smallest things,

the limp and dim quotidian—and grief, dripping

down the chins of everyone, like the juice

of the blackberries so ubiquitous here

this time of year a person could get sick of them.

A person could get sick of them, the days.
It will take me all of mine to learn to pray.
And then what? My parents risked the rest
of theirs to join us here. Oh, decadent
pandemic, where we feast on cardboard
and anxiety. Was it worth the risk? No way
to know. The question supposes scarcity,
a concept I have prayed to disbelieve.
It is August. I am tired of being brave.
I want to cling to the ones I love.
From the cages of our ribs, from the gates
of our seeing, we look out on all that is leaving
or has already left us. And we love each other
knowing this. Love is not innocuous.

Love is not innocuous. It runs

across the sullen fields where August burns

our bodies. Today I carried down the hill

the ashes of our dog. A month ago we carried

up his dying body. This wooden box, smaller

than the stuffed flamingo he tore apart yet kept

for years, is heavier than I'd expected but lighter

than seems fair. What happens to the rest of us,

and where? The scar on my arm where he clawed

against my bitter mercy has faded

and is almost gone. Now another day and we

are mocked by perfect weather, the neighbor

calling "come." We are left to hang

the rest of love, like laundry, in the sun.

August 16, 2020

Like laundry in the sun, our hanging hearts
might dry out, stiffen, fade, before all of this
is done. Chalk circles, six feet apart,
confine one person each: orientation week,
and the grass has never been so green.
Their pheromones, puzzled, mingle in the air,
and half a year's desire, muzzled,
bucks them there. In the office park tonight
deer nibble the topiary and down the street
in darkened yards campaign signs crouch
like small children sent outdoors
to study stars. Jupiter is so low and bright tonight
its reflection floats in my dark wine,
which I drink recklessly, inviting stains.

Inviting stain, inviting anything that might withstand

this rough erasure, I rush to work.

Graffiti on the utility box:

ARE YOU JUST GONNA SIT THERE AND WATCH

ME DIE, in purple magic marker. I go inside.

No cure for people dying forever.

"I'm sorry for your loss," I keep saying.

"I'm so sorry for your loss," I keep hearing

myself say. "Our bed," they called it. Now it's hers.

And his sneakers grow as empty as the hours,

then emptier. In their claw-foot tub, water seeks its most

lonely level: no one in it. We are left to perform

these badly written days—before an audience

of disembodied eyes—beneath a whiteout sky.

August 22, 2020

When the whiteout sky turned open-road blue

we drove north along the Hood Canal

to eat oysters, ostensibly—really

to trade one kind of sorrow for another

saltier one. We took a route we hadn't taken

through tunnels of spruce-dappled light, green

and gold meadows that swallowed their barns,

pleasure homes in the mudflats, clear-cuts

on the hillsides like the scars on a lover you turn from.

And though still only August, I felt that fine foil

of autumn on the air, which lent further flavor

to the oysters, like the taste of sight,

as I watched my daughter—not two years old—

slurp and smile, changed again by her delight.

Her delight defines a border softer
than the worn-out edge of the world and more
porous. Citrus-colored sunset. We tear old bread
to pieces and toss the pieces to the gulls.
Moments like this, when the galaxy grows
less callous, I know we contain within us
what overcomes us, that by which
we are swept away. She doesn't know this, doesn't need
to know to taste and see that all is always
coming to be. Unlike me, she plays above
the grim percussion of the morning news:
mutations in the virus—another chasm in our nation's
trust—a surplus of crumbs—the naming of the hurricanes
before they even come.

September 1, 2020

Each new hurricane that comes comes far from here

where the whale-deep waters swing, too far north

and cold to bear such storms. Instead, small rain

will fall for four months straight

and from the Narrows the insulated seals

will watch like dogs as we feed ourselves

upon the shore. One seal in particular

we have seen here, evening after evening—

he strikes his tail against the still

surface of the water, brassy with the setting sun.

He rings it like a higher drum as dark comes down.

Later, he'll wake us, splashing in the shallows.

The sound of thrashing as he feeds

will make it hard for us to fall back to sleep.

To fall back to sleep I try to remember

the names of forgotten major leaguers:

Tuffy Rhodes, Dickie Thon...

Morning finds me more than one

day older. I forfeit any sense of closure—

a bad trade for moving on. The day begins

invisibly, like a fire in the bio lab.

Six crows cut six crow-shaped holes in the sky.

Back in clinic, the waiting room is full of patients

and I am full of waiting rooms, and in each

a part of me is nodding off, or just forgetting

how to live. When all the sleep inside me wakes,

is that what dying is? Then someone calls my name

and I am startled from that dream into this one.

From that dream into this one

desire is moving through my life. Another summer

has singed the grass and we are waiting for the ferry

from the wrong side of Labor Day, our new kite

snagged high in the branches and my hand-me-down heart

sagging after too much wine. Yet my wife seems to be

growing wings, or becoming, at least, intimate with flight.

Like the fall-flowering crocuses in the orchard

near the harbor, she inhabits the secret of this season.

I watch her gather twigs and stems and braid them

for our daughter. She gleans a crown from fallen things.

And suddenly I remember a desire deeper than this dark

water, and bearing light like it—the same desire

flowing here, where we abandon the kite, and grow old together.

September 11, 2020

We grow old together, and life is endless in all ways

but one, the one in which plump summer shrivels up

and from vacant lots we hear the shock of wood

chopped, the construction—by division—of autumn's

tinder box. In the satellite image the plume of smoke

looks like a polluted sea, misplaced

on top of the city, some glitch in the digital map,

and here, within and under it, the sky is the absence

of sky—looking at it burns the eyes. The wildfires

have turned metaphor to fatal fact: our world

is burning. Subtract the sun. Paint high noon

a milquetoast dusk. You get the picture. Now picture fire

reflecting in the eyes of livestock left behind

in the evacuated town. Now picture it burned to the ground.

September 15, 2020

Each night burns to the ground. This morning I found

my car laminated with ash like contour lines

on an antique map. All the air purifiers

are on backorder, the smoke a bloated river

running sea to sea.

They were trying to tell us something, the trees,

before their whispers became the gasps of burning things.

Last time I saw the sky it was beautiful

the way a dumpster fire might be, before what you're seeing

has sunk in. We're sinking in, like pumpkins, hollowed

and aflame. It's not Halloween, but it looks the same.

We're in this together, and by *in* I mean *under*.

Make America over again. Teach it how to pray.

And by *pray*, I mean *listen*. There is always less to say.

There is always less to say. Like carrying
water, or a flame, I carry my silence,
and you carry yours. After the fires, finally,
tonight, the rain; and because it wasn't the taste
of apples and honey on our tongues but another
name for the dead, we followed—full of ruth,
bitter fruit—into the downpour we'd prayed for
and stood there until we were too drenched to distinguish
between bodies of water and bodies of air, ourselves
and our absent ones: gone, and everywhere.
And suddenly Xela wanted to make an altar,
too early, for Day of the Dead. So we did, in the pouring
down rain, strewing flowers and faces brightly framed
until who's to say if we were mourning or reveling?

September 28, 2020

Mourning or reveling, everything, all
at once, the walloping storm and the calm
that comes after it—I'll take all of it—
life—to be specific—until I die.
Some geese fly south across the blank-page sky,
prophetic hieroglyphics. *This ends well*
is what it means. I'm guessing. A roadside
puddle lets Oola dance on well spent clouds.
The neighborhood deer harvest deep russet
windfalls from the ground. Nothing is wasted,
love least of all. Past the tide flats, gulls feast
from mountains of trash. Driving to clinic,
day breaks its glass of light on the harbor
and I take it—like a chance—like a cure.

Acknowledgments

I am grateful to the editors of the following publications where some of these poems first appeared: *Poetry Northwest, Sixth Finch, Love's Executive Order, The American Literary Review, Plume,* and *Ploughshares*. I am especially grateful to Alice Quinn, who included two of the poems in her anthology, *Together in a Sudden Strangeness: America's Poets Respond to the Pandemic* (Knopf, 2020) and whose belief in this book has bolstered me.

Thank you to the friends who gave me the gift of close, critical readings of early drafts and helped to shape the book that is now in your hands: Bill Carty, Maria Chelko, Andrew Haley, Ben Jasnow, Nick Liptak, and Eleanor Martin.

Thank you to Curran Hatleberg for the image that graces the cover.

A number of other friends have encouraged me during the writing of this book and have been essential to its making: Luke Baker, Ariel Brantley-Daglish, Laura Brimo-Evin, Bheeshm Chaudhary, Liz Darhansoff, Zach Fox, Jeff Guay, Todd Gitlin, Tamie Herridge, Zannah Herridge-Meyer, Kathy Hourigan, Matthew Lippman, Keha McIlwaine, Dick Meyer, Michael Morse, Fernando Perez, Katie Peterson, Bob Scanlan, John Skoyles, Sarah Stickney, and Abe Streep.

Thank you to Askold Melnyczuk, Ezra Fox, and everyone at Arrowsmith Press for taking a chance on me. I am so proud to be in your company.

Thank you to Myron Glick for showing me how to be a doctor.

Thank you to all of my patients and colleagues at Sea Mar Community Health Center. It is my privilege to be there for and with you.

Thank you to my parents, Becky and Dan, for everything, actually.

Thank you to my sister, Lydia, whom I called every evening on my way home from clinic.

Finally, thank you to Xela, my first and best reader, my love.

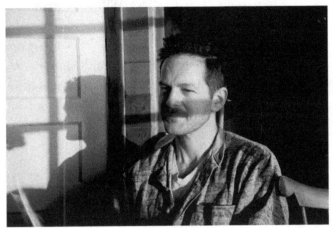

Photo by Lydia Okrent

John Okrent is a poet and a family doctor. His poetry has appeared in *Ploughshares, Plume, Poetry Northwest, Field,* and *The Seattle Times,* among other journals. He was chosen by Carl Phillips as the winner of the 2021 Jeff Marks Memorial Prize. Okrent works at a community health center in Tacoma, WA, where he lives with his wife and two young children in a fisherman's cabin on Puget Sound.

ARROWSMITH is named after the late William Arrowsmith, a renowned classics scholar, literary and film critic. General editor of thirty-three volumes of *The Greek Tragedy in New Translations*, he was also a brilliant translator of Eugenio Montale, Cesare Pavese, and others. Arrowsmith, who taught for years in Boston University's University Professors Program, championed not only the classics and the finest in contemporary literature, he was also passionate about the importance of recognizing the translator's role in bringing the original work to life in a new language.

Like the arrowsmith who turns his arrows straight and true,
a wise person makes his character straight and true.

— Buddha

Books by
ARROWSMITH
————PRESS————

Girls by Oksana Zabuzhko

Bula Matari/Smasher of Rocks by Tom Sleigh

This Carrying Life by Maureen McLane

Cries of Animal Dying by Lawrence Ferlinghetti

Animals in Wartime by Matiop Wal

Divided Mind by George Scialabba

The Jinn by Amira El-Zein

Bergstein edited by Askold Melnyczuk

Arrow Breaking Apart by Jason Shinder

Beyond Alchemy by Daniel Berrigan

Conscience, Consequence: Reflections on Father Daniel Berrigan edited by Askold Melnyczuk

Ric's Progress by Donald Hall

Return To The Sea by Etnairis Rivera

The Kingdom of His Will by Catherine Parnell

Eight Notes from the Blue Angel by Marjana Savka

Fifty-Two by Melissa Green

Music In—And On—The Air by Lloyd Schwartz

Magpiety by Melissa Green

Reality Hunger by William Pierce

Soundings: On The Poetry of Melissa Green edited by Sumita Chakraborty

The Corny Toys by Thomas Sayers Ellis

Black Ops by Martin Edmunds

Museum of Silence by Romeo Oriogun

City of Water by Mitch Manning

Passeggiate by Judith Baumel

Persephone Blues by Oksana Lutsyshyna

The Uncollected Delmore Schwartz edited by Ben Mazer

The Light Outside by George Kovach

The Blood of San Gennaro by Scott Harney edited by Megan Marshall

No Sign by Peter Balakian

Firebird by Kythe Heller

The Selected Poems of Oksana Zabuzhko edited by Askold Melnyczuk

The Age of Waiting by Douglas J. Penick

Manimal Woe by Fanny Howe

Crank Shaped Notes by Thomas Sayers Ellis

The Land of Mild Light by Rafael Cadenas edited by Nidia Hernández

The Silence of Your Name by Alexandra Marshall

Flame in a Stable by Martin Edmunds

Mrs. Schmetterling by Robin Davidson

CPSIA information can be obtained
at www.ICGtesting.com
Printed in the USA
JSHW041546260822
29715JS00002B/142